Live by Faith,

Live Healthy

and

Die Happy.

Medico-Scriptural Basis

Albert C. Lysinge, M.D.

Published by Teachersletters Publishing Services
Teachersletter@gmail.com, Douala.

Dedication

To *SETH MOKEBA LYSINGE* of Blessed Memory!

You keenly, anxiously and vainly waited for the completion of this book, but God decided to call you home, at the prime and vibrant age of 26, only few months to its final publication.

I can now testify from an eye-witness point of view that; "It is faith in God and hope for eternal life that makes death, or the loss of a loved one like you, peaceful, acceptable and bearable."

You will be **FOREVER IN OUR HEARTS**!

DADDY

Table of Content

ACKNOWLEDGEMENTS

I first of all give thanks to God the Almighty Father for His divine inspiration and grace to make this book a reality.

I immensely thank Miss Bame Juliet who did the typing of the manuscript and layout of the book, for her professionalism, patience and insight.

I am grateful to Rev Fr. Moses Tazoh for painstakingly proofreading the manuscript and making valuable suggestions towards improving the quality of the book.

Finally, I want to acknowledge in a very special way, my wife, Magdalene Limunga Lysinge and children: Brice Lifanje Lysinge, Edwin Teke Lysinge, Albert Chei Lysinge Jr, and Calmira Nalovah Lysinge, whose anxiety, enthusiasm and constant reminder kept me focused and steadfast on the task ahead of me. I'm sure I've lived up to all their expectations.

FOREWORD

LIVE WELL AND DIE HAPPY

You probably wonder why people in the Old Testament lived longer than the generations of today. Many of them lived beyond one hundred years. Dying before a hundred was an exception. Imagine that Moses was called to lead the Israelites out of Egypt when he was eighty. He performed that function actively for the next forty years without any major crisis or health hazards. "Moses was one hundred and twenty years old when he died; his sight was unimpaired and his vigor had not abated." (Deut. 34:7)

One would believe it is the same worry that led Dr. Lysinge to research and come up with some tips from Sacred Scripture, the medical field, and personal practical experience, that can enable us improve on our health. The secret is to be close to nature and stay far away from fast foods. A simple and moderate lifestyle and good eating habits will go a long way to keep body and soul together in good form. His caution on charlatans and false prophets is timely. Life is what you make it in truth.

What is even more remarkable about this much cherished informative book, on holistic wellbeing, is that the author has touched on many areas of health concerns, such as spirituality, medical science, physiotherapy, psychology, therapy, psychotherapy, and clinical psychology. Who would not like to live well and die happy? You would not regret giving yourself a good treat by devouring its content?

Rev. Fr. Moses Tazoh

PREFACE

God created humans to be like himself, in his own image and likeness (Gen 1:27). This divine privilege granted to us differentiates humans from other animal species, and naturally explains humankind's superiority over other animals. 'They will have power over the fish, the birds and all animals, domestic and wild, large and small (Gen 1:26[b])'

The spirit, mind and body are connected in a cycle and work in such a physiological manner that if the spirit is disturbed, the mind, through the brain, interprets the resulting imbalance. This imbalance or anomaly is in turn being transmitted through the nervous system as a signal to the body. The body in turn releases various chemical substances (hormones) that affect the organs and blood vessels such that poisonous substances (toxins) accumulate in the blood. This explains why a spiritual or emotional problem can affect the mind, part of the body or the whole body. This results in what is termed Psychosomatic Illnesses.

Medically, a spiritually and emotionally healthy person has a physically healthy body and any negative thoughts would have negative repercussions on the body.

This implies therefore that healing, through the mind, can be real and effective through positive thinking. Every human being, therefore, from the very essence of his/her inherent spirituality, has the power of thinking perfect health and obtaining nothing but perfect health in return. One cannot plant oranges and harvest apples!

Healing through positive thoughts can work harmoniously with medicine in a miraculous manner. The use of placebos in modern medicine illustrates this point. A placebo is a substance given to someone, making him/her think that it is a particular medicine, either to make him/her feel better, or to compare the effect of a particular drug when given to others in comparative studies. The placebo effect may turn out to be just as effective as or sometimes more effective than the real medication for that purpose. If you truly believe that the substance given you is a cure, then you will get what you believe and be completely cured.

Living by faith impacts positively on our health and healing. It also keeps us focused on eternity. The Scriptures say; "The person who is put right with God through faith shall live." (Rom 1:17)

The placebo effect in modern medicine is similar to the preponderant role played by faith in spiritual healing which is now gaining grounds in the world. Faith healing is gaining increasing and widespread popularity due to the fact that the majority of ailments and afflictions plaguing humanity are attributed to spiritual and emotional causes. This has also led to the proliferation of faith healers all over the world, some of whom are genuine and some fake. Notwithstanding, a clear distinction needs to be made between the true healer and the charlatan.

Alternative therapies, especially faith healing and natural remedies are rapidly overtaking Western medicine in recent times. This is because of the relative reliability and safety of natural products, coupled with the fact that modern medicine has its own flaws and limitations.

Natural or herbal medicine uses plants or plant products for healing, all of which are God's creation. At the beginning of creation, God gave specific dietary instructions to mankind, based on plants, as follows: *'I have provided all kinds of grain and all kinds of fruit for you to eat'* (Gen 1:29). If only mankind obeyed God's instructions by living on plant-based diet; made up of vegetables, fruits, nuts and whole grains, human beings would have been quite healthy, very strong and free from most diet-related diseases.

Besides the nutritional value of plants or plant products, mankind would have benefitted also from their natural medicinal or healing properties. These plants were all created by God and divinely designed both for feeding and for natural healing. The Psalmist declares, 'you make grass grow for the cattle and plants for human beings to use.' (Ps 104:14). Mankind, however, abandoned the use of plants and resorted to eating unhealthy foods and using artificial or synthetic products as medicine.

Amongst the many factors that can affect the health of humans significantly is lifestyle. Living on a proper diet, being physically active and engaging in adequate physical, aerobic and spiritual exercises would ensure good health and longevity.

Good health, healing, death and eternity are so interwoven that the one cannot be discussed or treated effectively without the others. They were all designed by God our creator, according to his will for mankind.

"For all things were created by him, and all things exist through him and for him. To God be the glory forever! Amen." (Rm 11:36)

This divinely motivated and inspirational book does not in any way contradict the principles of science and/or religion, but rather highlights the complete compliance or harmony between science and religion, or medicine and the Holy scriptures, for both are controlled and designed by God, who is Supreme, Omnipresent, Omniscient and Omnipotent.

For easy reading and a clear understanding of the related topics, this book has been divided into three main parts:

☐ **Part One** discusses living by faith and the place of faith healing in relation to Western medicine and natural therapy.

☐ **Part Two** focuses on healthy living with regard to proper feeding and adequate lifestyle.

☐ **Part Three** enunciates the outcome of living by faith until death, and obtaining a happy transition into eternity.

The book is intended as an invaluable life-guide and companion to all mankind, a great asset to every student, teacher, sportsman, sportswoman, believer, non-believer, 'man/woman of God', clergy, religious, the sick, the healthy, the poor, the rich, medical doctors and natural therapists. Finally, it is for posterity.

PART ONE:

LIVING BY FAITH

'Living by faith

isn't living

with certainty.

It's trusting God

in spite of unanswered

questions and

unresolved doubts.'

Rick Warrens

1:1   FAITH

'To have faith is to be sure of the things we hope for, to be certain of the things we cannot see.'

- Heb 11:1

Faith is simply defined as having great trust or confidence in something or someone. Common examples are the Muslim, Jewish, Buddhist or Christian faith. However, all the above-mentioned faithful have something in common. They all believe in the existence of a Supreme, Supernatural, Almighty or Spiritual being called Allah, Yahweh, Jehovah or God according to their respective religious leanings.

Being a convinced Christian, I will refer to that Supreme Being as God throughout this book, with due respect and no hurt or prejudice to non-Christian faithful. He is a God of mercy and love. He loved the world so much that he gave his only Son that everyone who believes in him may not perish, but may have eternal life. (Jn 32:27) He is the creator of all things and father of all believers and non-believers alike. He tells us, "I am the Lord, the God of all mankind. Nothing is too difficult for me." (Jer 32:27)

Some say that faith actually sees the invisible,

believes the incredible, and receives the impossible. Others have likened faith to WIFI; saying it is invisible yet has the power to connect you to what you need.

Amongst the biblical icons of faith, the Blessed Virgin Mary is considered by many as the supreme example of someone with profound faith. When the angel of the Lord announced to her that she would give birth to the Son of God, Mary answered; ***"I am the Lord's servant; may it happen to me as you have said.*** (Lk 1:38)." She accepted and welcomed God's word with faithful obedience, no matter how humanly impossible it seemed at that moment. Like Mary, we should always obey God and have trust in Him.

Abraham, the father of faith, was able to become a father even though he was too old and Sarah herself could not have children. He trusted God to keep his promise (Heb 11:11).

There is immeasurable power in faith, no matter the circumstances. This fact is clearly highlighted by our Lord Jesus Christ when he said to his disciples: "If you have faith as big as a mustard seed you can say to this hill, ***"Go from here to there!" and it will go. You could do anything!*** (Mt 17:20)." After much reflexion St. Anselm said that if we really want to know God as He is, then, the human intellect must seek a higher intellect called faith. Faith at this level seeks understanding (FIDES

QUAERENS INTELLECTUM). It is a great privilege and pride for me to maintain that "Fides Quaerens Intellectum" is the MOTTO of my ALMA MATER – St Joseph's College Sasse, BUEA.

The faith of those seeking breakthroughs, healing or deliverance should not be weakened if there is any delay in their requests being granted. Our God is a living God who is all loving, all merciful and all knowing.
He knows what is good for us and will grant it at his own appointed time. The popular adage "God's time is the best," re-iterates this point.

In the name of his Son, Jesus Christ, we can achieve or have anything. "For everyone who asks will receive, and everyone who seeks will find, and the door will be opened to those who knock. (Mtt 7:8)"

According to St. Augustine, faith is to believe what we do not see, and the reward of faith is to see what we believe. Therefore, no matter how long, or the form it takes, those who firmly believe will be rewarded accordingly.

1:2   FAITH HEALER

A faith healer is a person who cures sick people by using the power of prayer and belief. This is based on the belief that prayer, made in faith, will heal the sick person, the Lord will restore him to health, and the sins he committed will be forgiven (Jm 5:15). Our Lord Jesus Christ, who had both divine and human nature (both God and man), is believed to be the greatest, ultimate and genuine faith healer of all time.

There is a proliferation of faith healers in our world today with many of them heading famous and lucrative ministries that pull attractive crowds of people from all walks of life, irrespective of gender, creed, age or socio-economic status. In fact some of our local denominational churches are losing a significant number of Christians to these churches, synagogues or temples where prosperity messages are preached and instant miracles performed. These faith healers adorn themselves with titles such as Apostle, Evangelist, Disciple, Bishop, Prophet, Prophetess, etc. depending on their respective objectives, powers, background, location or socio-economic status. They are commonly or popularly referred to as "Men or Women of God." The troubling issue is that amongst them some are genuine and some fake. How can one then be able to draw a line or distinguish between a true faith healer and a false faith healer or charlatan?

1:2-1   TRUE VS FALSE FAITH HEALER

Our Lord Jesus warns; "Be on your guard against false prophets; they come to you looking like sheep on the outside, but on the inside they are really like wild wolves. You will know them by what they do. Thorn bushes do not bear grapes, and briars do not bear figs. A healthy tree bears good fruit, but a poor tree bears bad fruit. And any tree that does not bear good fruit will be cut down and thrown in the fire. So then you will know the false prophets by what they do." (Mtt 7:15-20)

The power and authority to heal spiritually must come from God. We learn that Jesus Christ called his twelve disciples together and gave them authority to drive out evil spirits and to heal every disease and every sickness (Mtt 10:1). A genuine man / woman of God claiming to heal spiritually must acknowledge, project and portray Jesus Christ as the ultimate healer and master. When the Apostle Peter made a paralyzed man to walk he did not claim the glory, instead he said; "Jesus Christ makes you well." (Act 9:34). It is written that, "God raised him to the highest place above and gave him the name greater than any other name. And so in honour of the name of Jesus all beings in heaven, on earth and in the world below will fall on their knees and all will openly proclaim that Jesus Christ is Lord, to the glory of God the Father."(Phil 2:9-11).

In addition to a very profound and unwavering faith, a true faith healer must empower and spiritually nourish himself or herself always through prayer and fasting to enable him / her succeed in healing and deliverance. He / she must not rely on his / her own ability, intelligence or spiritual powers. We read how Jesus, who is Lord and master, often withdrew to a lonely place to pray. And he fasted for forty days and forty nights (Mtt 4:2) before beginning his earthly ministry. This shows the importance of prayer and fasting as a means of spiritual nourishment and empowerment as evidenced by the Son of God himself.

A true faith healer must not seek powers from other gods. Many false healers practise magical acts, as opposed to the mystical acts attributed to Jesus. The psalmist cautions. "The gods of the nations are made of silver and gold; they are formed by human hands. They have mouths but cannot speak, and eyes but cannot see. They have ears but cannot hear; they are not even able to breathe. May all who made them and who trust in them become like the idols they have made!" (Ps 135:15-18)

The true "man / woman of God" should be humble and focused on God's kingdom, rather than on the world. Their minds should not be set mainly on earthly things and they should shun arrogant display of wealth or living in affluence. Some live in heavily guarded and expensive homes, move in a convoy of expensive cars with guards, have multiple and huge bank accounts, have private jets and yachts and multiple concubines etc. Vanity of vanities, says the preacher, vanity of vanities! All is vanity (Eccl 1:2). The first book of Timothy tells us that;

'whoever teaches a different doctrine and does not agree with the true words of our Lord Jesus Christ, and with the teaching of our religion, is swollen with pride and knows nothing........ They think that religion is a way to become rich' (1 Tim 6:3-5). These false 'men/women' of God make religion a means of livelihood, thus enriching themselves after the sweat of the labour of their followers.

Like the prophets of old, genuine prophets should be humble and selfless messengers who act or speak on God's behalf, and should focus their gaze on God's kingdom rather than on themselves or earthly possessions. It is said that, "............ your Father in heaven knows that you need all these things. Instead, be concerned above everything else with the kingdom of God and with what he requires of you, and he will provide you with all these things." (Mtt 6:32^b-33)

A true faith healer should always follow in the footsteps and teachings of Christ. Instead of preaching the gospel as it is, some fake healers would rather tell you what you would like to hear, in defiance of the truth. Nothing makes the Lord happier than to hear that his children live in the truth (3 Jn: 4).

The true faith healer doesn't need to request any form of remuneration, whether cash or kind, as a prerequisite for healing or deliverance. Jesus instructed his disciples to, ***"Heal the sick, bring the dead back to life, heal those who suffer from dreaded skin diseases and*** *drive out demons. You have received without paying; so give without being paid*" (Mtt 10:8). It is commonplace to see around us people, especially women, who offer their salaries, cars, land and, in some cases, their virginity to some fake and delinquent faith healers, under the guise of sowing seeds, in return for certain favours, such as having a suitor, employment, promotion, a VISA, deliverance, healing, exam success, etc. A friend of mine once made the pertinent remark that, while Jesus fed thousands of destitute and hungry people, some "men / women of God" are shamelessly being fed and financially empowered by thousands of desperate, sick and poor people in need of prosperity messages and instant solutions to their predicaments. This fosters "the rich get richer and the poor get poorer" syndrome, thus causing untold and widespread misery or hardship to mankind in general, and to the poor, suffering humanity in particular. A true faith healer doesn't need to advertise his healing, deliverance, prophecy or miracle sessions. Today we see them advertising on both conventional and social media. Some go as far as announcing and predicting the number and type of miracles to be performed on the D-Day. Our Lord Jesus after healing two blind men, told them not to tell anyone (Mtt 2:30). This was the messianic secret as most people did not believe that Jesus was the Messiah and Saviour. Despite this warning the news still spread because anything done in the Spirit of God cannot be hidden or concealed. Genuine faith healers should therefore function or act in spirit and in truth, and leave the rest to God. News about their good works or actions would eventually spread far and wide without any intended, wilful or dramatized publicity. All flyers or stickers with biblical quotations and verses, portraits, amulets, anointing oils or water, must clearly reflect Jesus Christ the healer, deliverer, protector, provider and saviour. It is despicable for these faith healers to provide and sell portraits and other articles carrying their personal pictures or caption to their followers, who end up idolizing and worshipping them. They are mere messengers of the master and not vice versa. We must give honour to whom honour is due; for it is written, "Everything you do or say, then, should be done in the name of the Lord Jesus, as you give thanks through him to God the Father" (Col 3:17).

A true faith healer shouldn't dwell only on prosperity messages and discard all possibilities of suffering, ill – health, other afflictions and even death. They emit ridiculous, unrealistic and far–fetched utterances like; sickness is not your portion, failure is not your portion, poverty is not your portion, and even death is not your portion. Where have they put the will and plan of God for mankind in general, and the individual in particular? There is no Christianity without the cross, and every human being must be willing and prepared always to accept and carry his / her cross accordingly, in all circumstances and at all times. Jesus said, "If any man would come after me, let him deny himself and take up his cross daily and follow me" (Lk 9:23). He, the Son of God, was misunderstood, accused, rejected, persecuted, tortured, crucified and died a shameful death on a tree. How come we, mere humans, would expect to be dissociated and spared from the ups and downs of life. No matter how prayerful, pious or faithful we are, the good and merciful God will not always grant our requests or needs according to our desires, but He will surely grant what is good for us according to his will and at his own appointed time. May the will of God be manifested in our lives – Amen.

A genuine faith healer doesn't indulge in blackmail, gossip, defamation or carry out hate speech against a fellow faith healer or rival ministry. This would cause unhealthy competition and rivalry amongst existing ministries and ministers, and would bring about confusion and division amongst Christians or followers. Apostle Paul warns; "I urge you my brothers and sisters: watch out for those who cause divisions and upset people's faith and go against the teaching which you have received. Keep away from them! For those who do such things are not serving Christ our Lord, but their own appetite. "By their fine words and flattering speech they deceive innocent people" (Rom 16:17-18).

Our Lord Jesus preached the appearance of false prophets and warned us to be on our guard; "for false Messiahs and false prophets will appear. They will perform miracles and wonders in order to deceive even God's chosen people, if possible. Be on your guard! I have told you everything before the time comes "(Mk 13:22-23). The time is here already, with the proliferation of these prophets and prophetesses in our communities and neighbourhoods. They function with unrepentant impunity and ferocious audacity, at times under the protection and connivance of some top administrative or security officials. Some even do it as a big business venture in partnership with people of known integrity and affluence in the society or in partnership with other business magnets. Some have branches or networks across national frontiers and across the globe. Some are committing extensive and lamentable atrocities and crimes which are now being exposed and condemned, and some governments have started pursuing, persecuting or banishing them from their territories.

The fate of the self-styled, false prophet is clearly documented: 'But the prophet who presumes to say in my name a thing I have not commanded him to say or who speaks in the name of other gods, that prophet shall die' (Deut 18:20).

It must be emphasized, however, that the existence of honest and genuine faith healers cannot be ruled out, and the few good seeds should not be condemned, criticised or chastised alongside the bad seeds. These spiritually gifted and trustworthy messengers of God sometimes work in collaboration with medical doctors and natural therapists for better diagnosis, management and holistic treatment of certain patients. It is worth noting that faith healing is not the monopoly or preserve of a particular denomination, group of persons or individual. The Spirit of God manifests in anyone who believes in Him. The Apostle John is said to have reported to Jesus that a man who did not belong to their group was driving out demons in Jesus' name, and Jesus replied; 'Do not try to stop him because no one who performs a miracle in my name will be able soon afterwards to say evil things about me. For whoever is not against us is for us (Mk 9:39-40)."

Whether fake or genuine, these faith healers will meet their fate accordingly. The scripture says, "Do not deceive yourselves; no one makes a fool of God. A person will reap exactly what he sows. If he sows in the field of his natural desires, from it he will gather the harvest of death; if he sows in the field of the Spirit, from the spirit he will gather the harvest of eternal life" (Gal 6:7-8)

To all those seeking faith healing, deliverance or breakthroughs, these guidelines should serve as an eye opener that will help them make a clear distinction between a true and a false faith healer.

I admonish all those who are already well rooted in

a particular healing ministry or who are ardent followers of a particular prophet or prophetess to revisit their decision or stance before continuing in that fellowship.

Finally, to all the well-established, famous, affluent, celebrated or aspiring "men / women of God," I make a clarion call for an examination of conscience on whether they are serving God or their earthly desires and passions. *"**No one can serve two masters**! (Mtt 6:24)"* God will reward or punish each person according to whether he / she is glorifying Him or whether it is for his / her personal glorification. The choice is yours!

1:3   FAITH HEALING

Faith healing is the act of healing by faith. It may involve the faith of the healer, the faith of the sick or afflicted person, or the faith of any third party accompanying the patient.

The Lord Jesus said; "If you ask me for anything in my name, I will do it" (Jn 14:14). Any person or group of persons can effectively intercede for anyone to be healed or delivered in the name of Jesus.

Faith healing actually involves the practice of prayer and some gestures, such as laying of hands, that are believed, be some Christians, to elicit divine intervention in spiritual and physical healing. The use of faith healing to heal human illness dates back thousands of years in history. Evidence of its use in ancient Egypt is found in the Ebers Papyrus dated around 1552BC.

The popular adage, *"doctors treat and Jesus heals,"* reminds us of the fact that, although we seek medical attention and treatment from medical doctors or natural therapists, it is the Lord who does the ultimate and definitive healing. He said to the Israelites; "If you will obey me completely by doing what I consider right and by keeping my commandments, I will not punish you with any of the diseases that I brought on the Egyptians. *I am the Lord the one who heals you*" (Ex 15:26)

Prophet Jeremiah asked for healing from the Lord, trusting and believing that the Lord would grant him a complete and holistic healing; "Lord heal me and I will be completely well .... (Jer 17:14)".

Faith has an undisputed role to play in the treatment and healing of the mind and soul, but also of the underlying or root cause of the disease affecting the body. The Lord heals the broken – hearted and bandages their wounds (Ps 147:3).

Sin can greatly impair faith healing, thus it is imperative that one should acknowledge one's sins and repent before seeking healing or deliverance. The psalmist says; "He will forgive all my sins and heal my diseases."

(Ps 103:3).

God created man and the universe in such a way that there is an ecological balance between humans, plants, animals and every other thing that exists in the world. Any natural or man – made disruption of this balance would cause an unpleasant, unnatural and destructive imbalance that would adversely affect our health and consequently reduce our lifespan. This confirms the fact that humans cannot be healthy or well in an unhealthy or sick environment. An unhealthy environment would sooner or later cause ecological disaster on a large scale. This is exactly what happened with the outburst, spread and extensive damage caused by the scary COVID – 19 pandemic all over the world. The solution to societal ills today, such as greed, corruption, tribalism, occultism, marginalization, witchcraft, terrorism, wars, genocide, sexual/drug abuse, homosexuality, cannibalism, xenophobia, etc. can only be sought through spiritual healing or cleansing that encompasses humans and their habitat at large. The Lord says, "I will heal this city and its people and restore them to health. I will show them abundant peace and security" (Jer 33:6-7). Every land that has been desecrated by bloodshed, occultic practices or generational curses must be healed spiritually for mankind to be truly healed. This type of holistic healing can only be achieved if we repent and turn to the Lord in deep faith and total trust.

We read how people who had demons in them were brought to Jesus and he drove out the evil spirits with a word and healed all who were sick. He did this to make what the prophet Isaiah had said come true, "He himself took our sickness and carried away our diseases" (Mtt 8:16-17). It was because of our sins that he was wounded, and beaten because of the evil we did. And that we are healed by the punishment he suffered, and made whole by the blows he received (1s 53:5). Jesus is therefore the undisputed and divine healer. He is also master of all things including evil spirits and natural disasters. No wonder the disciples asked one another in utter dismay after he had calmed the storm: "Who is this man? Even the wind and the waves obey Him!" (Mk 4:41)

The faith of the people of Gennesaret is worth emulating. They accepted, trusted and believed in Jesus and begged him to let those who were sick to at least touch the edge of his cloak; and all who touched it were made well (Mtt 14:36).

The Canaanite woman cried out and begged Jesus to have mercy on her and heal her daughter who had a demon, and was in a terrible state. Despite the fact that Jesus told her that it wasn't right to take the children's food and throw it to the dogs, she persisted and answered

Jesus that it was true what he said but even the dogs ate the left overs that fell from the master's table. Jesus, overwhelmed by her response and unwavering faith, answered her, ***"You are a woman of great faith! What you want will be done for you."*** And at that very moment her daughter was said to be healed (Mtt 15:22-28). This woman teaches us the importance of humility and perseverance in faith when faced with problems and challenges.

The woman with the issue of blood had suffered for twelve years consulting many doctors and spending all her money to no avail. When she heard about Jesus she infiltrated the crowd behind him, saying to herself, "If I just touch his cloak, I will get well." She touched his cloak and her bleeding stopped instantly. Jesus, realising that power had gone out of him, turned round and asked; "Who touched my clothes?" when the woman realised what had happened to her, she came out trembling with fear, knelt at Jesus' feet and told him the whole truth. Jesus said to her, ***"My daughter, your faith has made you well. Go in peace, and be healed of your trouble."*** (Mtt 5:25-34). This woman's immense faith, courage and truthfulness made her well.

King Hezekiah cried out to the Lord in prayer when he was ill, and the Lord sent prophet Isaiah to go and say to him, "I the Lord, the God of your ancestor David, have heard your prayer and seen your tears, I will heal you." (2kg 20:4-5). The lesson here is that whenever we are sick or afflicted, we should cry out to the Lord in prayer and in faith, and the Lord will either intervene directly to solve our problem or use messengers such as faith healers, medical doctors or natural therapists to heal us, or transmit the assurance of his divine healing and deliverance to us just as he sent prophet Isaiah to King Hezekiah.

Also, when you pray and don't have what you want, it is because you have not prayed enough or properly. And when you ask, and you do not receive, it is because your motives are bad; you ask for things to use for your own pleasures (Jas 4:3).

The story is told of the Roman officer who wanted Jesus to heal his sick servant. He told his friends that he didn't deserve to have Jesus enter his house, and that he was not also worthy to go to Jesus in person. But, that Jesus should just give an order and his servant would be healed. On hearing this Jesus, surprised, turned round and said to the crowd following him; "I tell you, I have never found faith like this, not even in Israel! (Lk 7:9)." Despite his position of authority and command, the officer acknowledged, in all humility, his unworthiness or emptiness before Christ and fervently believed that just a word from the Lord would suffice in healing his servant, without even seeing or touching him. Like the officer, when requesting faith healing, we must have a childlike trust and belief in our Lord and master Jesus Christ. It is clearly stated that whoever believes in him will not be disappointed (Rm 10:11).

Faith is said to come from hearing the message, and the message comes through preaching Christ (Rm 10:17)

The Holy Spirit instructs us: "If only you would listen to him today! Do not harden your hearts, as at the rebellion, as at the time of testing in the desert, when your ancestors challenged me." (Heb 3:7-8). Our generation has no valid excuse for not believing the good news message. Its spread has been greatly facilitated by the availability and accessibility of conventional and social media. But we seem to be carried away by earthly desires such as sexual immorality, indecency, lust, evil passions and greed. Because of such things, God's anger will come upon those who do not obey him (Col 3:5-6). It is only by opening up to receiving and accepting the message, and by having profound faith and childlike trust or belief in Jesus, that we can be beneficiaries of his mercy and obtain complete physical and spiritual healing or deliverance.

Eloquent testimony of faith healing is when the Lord asked Moses to make a bronze serpent and lift it up on a standard so that anyone bitten by a venomous snake, and who looked at it, would be healed and find life again. In the same way the Son of man must be lifted up so that everyone who believes in him may have eternal life. For God so loved the world that he gave his only Son, so that everyone who believes in him may not die but have eternal life (Jn 3:16). In modern medicine, the serpent on a standard is the symbol attributed to medical doctors and is usually affixed to the front or / and rear windscreens of their vehicles. This shows the undisputed and inalienable life – long and divine relationship between medicine and religion. It also shows the preponderant role played by faith healing in the treatment of most ailments or afflictions plaguing humanity.

The role of faith in the prevention of many illnesses or afflictions cannot be overlooked. By causing the prevention or absence of these ailments faith can significantly reduce hospital visits or expenses, and can also free one from the unpleasant side effects or complications associated with the consumption of synthetic drugs when one is sick. He (the Lord) will keep you safe from hidden dangers and from all deadly diseases (Ps 91:1-3). Most psychosomatic illnesses would be prevented if we have trust in God and avoid fear or anxiety. The phrases: 'Do not be afraid or fear not' are so important that they appear 365 times in the Bible, giving an average of about once every day in our lives. Those who wait patiently on the Lord in faith and in belief would be free from many ailments and afflictions. If couples with infertility problems, for example, persist in prayer, obey God's commandments and persevere in their faith, the Lord would eventually grant them fruit of the womb, no matter how long it would take. That was Zechariah and Elisabeth's situation. The angel of the Lord appeared to him and said, "Don't be afraid, Zechariah! God has heard your prayer, and your wife Elizabeth will bear you a son. You are to name him John." (Lk 1:13). It is also written that it was faith that made Abraham able to become a father, even though he was too old and Sarah herself could not have children. He trusted God to keep his promise (Heb 11:11). The psalmist states that God honours the childless wife in her home and he makes her happy by giving her children (Ps 11:9).

Infertile or sterile couples should refrain from consulting witchdoctors in search of fruit of the womb. Children issuing from such obscure sources are of doubtful origin and would tend to bring untold and inexplicable misery to the entire family, sooner or later. Those with infertility problems, if they continue to have faith in God and obey his commandments, would have their condition turned around in their favour and would be blessed with healthy, pretty and protected children, no matter how long it would take to have them. The scriptures reassure us that, "If only you had listened to my commands! Then blessings would have flowed for you like a stream that never goes dry! Victory would have come to you like the waves that roll on the shore. Your descendants would be as numerous as grains of sand, and I would have made sure they were never destroyed" (Is 48:18)

Faith therefore plays an indispensable role in the prevention or reversal of certain illnesses or related conditions.

1:4 MODERN MEDICINE VS NATURAL THERAPY

Nowadays faith healing and natural remedies are rapidly overtaking modern medicine. This is even more evident with the appearance of the controversial COVID-19 deadly pandemic, especially as African and Asian countries have registered more successes in its treatment with natural or herbal medicines than with modern medicine.

Generally, therapies and approaches to health and healing that are not considered parts of conventional, evidence –based (western) medicine are referred to as Complementary and Alternative Medicine (CAM). It is also referred to by others as "Integrative" medicine.

1:4 – 1 NATURAL REMEDIES

Natural or herbal medicine uses plant-based substances as the basis for treatment. It is believed to be the oldest and still the most widely used system of medicine in the world. According to WHO, an estimated 80% of people around the world use herbal medicine.

It uses fresh parts of plants, such as their roots, leaves, fruits, flowers, backs, seeds, nuts and grains. It may also be available as various preparations, such as herbal teas, alcoholic extracts, non-alcoholic glycerine extracts, powders, tablets, capsules and topical preparations (creams, ointments, liniments, pessaries, infused oils, poultices and compresses).

So far, natural remedies have proved to be healthy, efficacious, more beneficial and less harmful to humans than artificial or synthetic products. Notwithstanding, due to the massive presence of impudent herbal therapists or quack native doctors, the safety of herbal medicine cannot be guaranteed 100 per cent; mainly due to factors related to poor hygiene and improper dosage.

Contrary to some baseless, misguided and futile propaganda, natural or herbal remedies are neither against religion nor science. The scriptures tell us that the trees will provide food and their leaves will be used for healing (Ez 47:12)

Certified or licensed natural therapists should not

be confused with witch doctors, who use traditional magic or invoke evil spirits as part of their treatment. Some would make absurd requests before instituting treatment, such as providing a spotless white owl, the tooth of a spider, the claws of a lion or the genitals of a virgin etc. Such absurd practices are unhealthy, doubtful, dangerous and often with strings attached. It is said that with the devil there is no free gift.

David Avocado Wolfe studied the progress and development of medical practice, faith healing and natural therapy over the past 4000 years and came up with the following:

2000BC: Here, eat this Root

1000AD: That Root is Heathen! Here say this Prayer.

1865AD: That Prayer is superstition! Here drink this Portion.

1935AD: That Portion is Snake Oil! Here swallow this Pill.

1975AD: That Pill is ineffective! Here take this Antibiotic.

2000AD: That Antibiotic is poison! Here eat this Root.

Over a period of 4000 years, mankind moved from using natural remedies (Root), to spiritual or faith healing

(Prayer), then to the Pill and Antibiotic (Orthodox / Western Medicine) and has finally gone back to the Root (natural therapy). Therefore, it took about 4000 years for mankind to understand and learn (by experience) that natural remedies, as recommended by God, are healthier and more efficacious to humans than the portion, the pill and the antibiotic.

The Scripture says, "People of Egypt, go to GILEAD and look for medicine! All your medicine has proved useless; nothing can heal you" (Jer 46:11). It should be noted that GILEAD is a region east of the Jordan, famous for its medicinal plants. This was a divine recommendation for God's children to drop conventional therapy that was not helping them, and move towards natural therapy which is plant – based.

1.4-2 LIMITATIONS AND FLAWS IN MODERN MEDICINE

Some Remedies are Worse than the disease'

- **Pubilius Syrus.**

Modern medicine uses a scientific approach that ignores entire methods of therapy or other medical systems that do not align with this approach or model. Medical practitioners function within the limits of knowledge made available to them by modern medical and scientific research. Instead of treating the underlying or root causes of disease, medical doctors most often manage symptoms. This type of palliative therapy only makes the problem seem less serious; often by reducing pain, without curing the cause of the pain, the disease itself, or other associated signs and symptoms.

Pharmaceutical industries form an integral part of modern medicine and play a role in the management and treatment of certain diseases, within the limits of modern scientific research and latest discoveries. Drugs that are being sold or publicized today may be rejected or withdrawn from the market tomorrow, either because of their toxicity to humans or because of their increased ineffectiveness due to resistance. Also, pharmaceutical industries are out to do big business and would not in any way compromise their profits. In many countries the availability, acceptance and success of a particular drug depends on the bargaining power of the pharmaceutical industry officials, and the dividends put at the disposal of the authorities of those countries.

These pharmaceutical industries are indispensable in the sense that modern medicine would have been incomplete, inconceivable and impracticable without their products or drugs. This is because they both interrelate and form an integral part of one another.

The proliferation of unqualified medical personnel or quack doctors, working in clandestine health facilities or clinics in our communities, is doing a lot of damage to the population. It is commonplace to see nurses who own private clinics where they themselves work as both medical director and general practitioner. Many are the laboratory technicians who carry out general consultation, management and treatment of patients, or even minor surgery and hospitalisation. Some even go as far as selling drugs to the public in general. Even qualified medical doctors and specialists are not spared, as dishonesty and indiscriminate quest for money has eaten deep into the fabrics of their medical practice. In fact medical malpractice has resulted in uncountable and unaccountable number of deaths and, most often, the perpetrators of this criminal or "jungle" medical practice get away with it. In many cases, the "Hippocratic" oath becomes the "hypocritical" oath in action.

The above–mentioned short comings, together with the unpleasant or hazardous side-effects of some synthetic drugs, have contributed significantly to the failures and flaws attributed to modern medicine, with a corresponding increase in mortality rate in our communities.

A great doctor kills more than a great general.

- G.W. Leibniz

The failures and flaws, compounded by the increase in mortality rates in the world in general, have caused the credibility, dependence and hope that mankind had for Western medicine to dwindle drastically.

Despite the increase and availability of qualified medical personnel, specialists, improved health facilities or referral hospitals, and the recent advances made in scientific research, there are still a lot of unanswered questions and hopeless situations in modern medical practice. This was acknowledged by a great physician as follows:

"From inability to let well alone, from too much zeal for the new, and contempt for what is old, from putting knowledge before wisdom, science before art, and cleverness before common sense, from treating patients as cases and from making the cure of the disease more grievous than the endurance of the same, good Lord deliver us."

Sir Robert Hutchinson(1870-1960).

Firstly, he acknowledged in all humility, the bitter truth that medical doctors do aggravate or make worse the patient's condition in many cases. Secondly, he brings to light the uneasy fact that doctors often treat the disease and not the patient per se, implying that they don't treat the human body as an integrated whole. The mind and body are thus seen as separate, independent entities, and emotions are often neglected or completely ignored.

Moliere also remarked: "Nearly all men die of their medicines and not of their illnesses."

Modern medicine doesn't consider the human being as part of nature, and how things happening in nature or the environment may affect the human being health-wise.

Doctors completely ignore the fact that the body has a self-healing capacity. They go ahead and prescribe drugs for every situation, complaint or every sign and symptom, instead of seeking ways of boosting that self-healing capacity.

The importance of proper diet and life-style on health is also often downplayed, and the use of natural supplements to optimize health is overlooked in most cases.

The choice of therapy at any given moment, whether by faith healing, natural therapy or modern medical treatment should take into consideration the safety, risk and benefits to the human body as a whole, as well as its relationship to nature or the environment. This is the proper, holistic approach to be adopted by all humans for optimum health and healing.

1.4-3 THE UPSIDE OF MODERN MEDICINE.

Notwithstanding the aforementioned pitfalls and limitations, modern medicine has its own merits that are deserving of praise and should not be overlooked.

A- Regular Medical Check-up:

+Laboratory Investigations: Blood sugar levels;Triglycerides and Cholesterol levels; Complete Blood Count (CBC).

+ Blood Pressure Measurement.

+Routine Antenatal tests (Pregnant women).This must be done for foetal and maternal well-being and include: Weight and Height measurements done at the booking appointment; Blood Pressure measurement; Laboratory Investigations: Urine and Blood tests (blood type and Rhesus factor); Ultrasound Scans: at the first, second and third trimesters (normally an average of three times).

+Cancer Screening Tests: especially for Breast cancer, Cervical cancer, Prostate cancer, Lung cancer, POLYPS and Colorectal cancer.

The importance of regular medical checks is that early diagnosis leads to a more successful, less complicated and cost-effective management or treatment. This is especially true for cancers that are detected early.

B- Emergency Surgery:

Modern medicine takes care of live-saving surgical procedures which Alternative medicine cannot handle promptly or incisively. However, faith healing and natural remedies should always accompany such procedures for complete physical and spiritual recovery to be assured(holistic healing).Examples are: Colectomy- done for complete bowel obstruction or uncontrolled bleeding; Small bowel resection- done for diseased or blocked small bowel; Cholecystectomy- done for Gallstones in the Gallbladder; Stomach perforation due to ulcers; Appendicectomy- for an infected Appendix; Removal of Abdominal Adhesions as a result of the twisting and pulling within small or large intestines; Traumatic Injuries depending on the organ or gravity ,especially after a road traffic accident(RTA); C-section-done where delivery through the vaginal route would put the baby or mother at risk, thus preventing maternal or foetal deaths.

1.4-4 HOLISTIC HEALING

The holistic doctor or therapist is different from the conventional doctor in the sense that he/she cares for the general well-being rather than just trying to address a specific biological issue. Holistic healthcare covers the whole person by considering his/her mental, social, physical and spiritual needs. It also involves the emotional and environmental aspects. It is based on the premise that one's overall health is being affected by all those aspects, and presenting an illness in one aspect affects the other aspects. They should not be handled in isolation; a balance must be sought between all these dimensions for proper healing.

PART TWO

HEALTHY LIVING

35

HEALTHY CITIZENS ARE THE GREATEST ASSET

ANY COUNTRY CAN HAVE'.

- Winston Churchill

2.1 INTRODUCTION

At the beginning, when God created the world, he gave a clear dietary instruction to mankind:

'I have provided all kinds of grain and all kinds of fruits for you to eat'. (Gen 1:29)

Today, mankind has deviated from this divine dietary prescription with scornful impunity. We employ all sorts of methods in cooking the food we eat, such as firewood, charcoal, kerosene, gas, electricity, microwave, etc. We don't even take into consideration the potential hazards or toxicity associated with these various methods of cooking.

Some of the pots we us in cooking release carcinogenic (cancer-causing) particles that dissolve in the food in the process. Also, prolonged cooking or excessive heating destroys or alters the composition of the useful components or nutrients of most basic foodstuffs.

Some people eat a lot of processed or junk foods that cause poor health or related illnesses, especially when eaten in large amounts or over a long period.

God created some animals to be herbivorous (feeding only on plants), some to be carnivorous (flesh eaters only) and humans to be omnivorous (feeding on both plants and flesh). Incidentally the flagrant misuse of this dietary privilege or flexibility is the cause of most of mankind's health problems, with a consequent reduction in lifespan. It is therefore natural and obvious that a lion that feeds only on grass will not survive, a goat that feeds only on flesh will not thrive, and a human being who feeds on both grass and flesh in an uncontrolled, unbalanced and abusive manner will not be in good health.

Consuming more of plant products and less of flesh and its related products would cause humans to be stronger, healthier and to have an increase in lifespan.

The story is told of Daniel who went to the guard whom Ashpenaz had placed in charge of him and his three friends, and requested that he should test them for 10days, by giving them only vegetables to eat and water to drink. Then he should compare them with the young men who were eating the royal food, and then base his arguments on how they look. After ten days of trial, Daniel and his three friends who were put on vegetable diet and water looked healthier and stronger than all the young men who had been eating royal food (Daniel 1:11-15).This story of Daniel as narrated by the book of wisdom is eloquent testimony to the fact that humans can be very strong and healthy by living only on vegetables and water.

Besides a proper diet and adequate water intake, we're going to examine other related factors, mainly lifestyle, that plays a significant role in improving our health.

'Life is like a server. What you get out of it depends on what you put in.'

- Tom Lehrer

In reality, it is far easier to preserve health than to cure the disease.

2.2   HEALTHY EATING

'Our food should be our medicine, and our medicine should be our food.'

- Hippocrates (father of medicine)

Nature operates in such a way that if you don't eat your food as your medicine, you'd have to eat medicine as food. Ironically or sadly enough, many people compromise their health by eating in an unhealthy manner. Such people focus more on swelling their bank accounts or amassing property. They forget too often to realise that in case they fall sick, more money will be spent on drugs or other medical bills, and their time will be wasted for numerous hospital visits. They may even end up dying, leaving all their property and huge bank accounts to be squandered or plundered by family members or, worse still, unknown persons.

One of my closest friends once told me that whatever goes into your stomach in the form of food or drink is the only thing that belongs to you alone. I totally agree with his assertion.

A balanced diet is a combination of the correct types and amounts of food.

Carbohydrates are the main fuels of the body. It is transformed into glucose, which in turn is burnt to produce calories. High calorie foods should be restricted. Refined carbohydrates can be harmful because much fibre has been removed. They are also low in nutrients (empty calories) and are linked to overeating and many other diseases.

Added sugar foods and beverages should be minimised or avoided. They may cause various diseases such as obesity, type 2 diabetes, heart disease and many forms of cancer.

Fats are a rich source of energy. Excessive fats should be limited, taking into consideration the fact that the human body needs some amount of good fats. Excess fats not used for energy is deposited in the tissues in the form of body fat.

Because of their effects in the diet, unsaturated fats (monounsaturated and poly-unsaturated) are often referred to as good fats. Extra virgin olive oil is believed to be the healthiest fat on earth. It is very high in monounsaturated fats and contains a modest amount of vitamins E and K. It lowers blood pressure thus decreases the risk of cardio-vascular diseases. Other sources of monounsaturated fats are avocados, almonds, cashews, peanuts, etc. These fats can also be obtained from cooking oils produced from plants or seeds such as canola, peanut, olive, soybean, sesame and sunflower.

Polyunsaturated fats are also good but should be consumed in smaller quantities than monounsaturated fats. They can be obtained from walnuts, flaxseeds or corn oil, etc. Other sources are the salmon, herring and colbacore tuna fishes.

These good fats are known to reduce bad cholesterol in the blood (LDL Cholesterol), thus reduce the risk of heart disease. Fats from the above sources should be consumed instead of animal fats found in bacon, butter or lard. Animal fats produce carcinogenic substances amongst others.

Hidden fats found in canned or prepared foods such as French fries, pastries, etc. should also be avoided. Processed and junk foods lead to weight gain and many unpleasant ailments because they are known to have toxic fats, depleted flours, increased sugar, salt and food additives and preserves.

Proteins are used mainly for growth and repair of body tissues. They are transformed into amino acids which, when in excess, are burned to produce energy.

Minerals (trace elements) and vitamins are indispensable, in small amounts, for the functioning of the human body. They enable and facilitate the numerous chemical transformations which take place in the human cells.

The correct ratio of carbohydrates, fats, proteins, vitamins, minerals and water forms 'an adequate diet' that allows the human being to carry out the desired functions of reproduction, growth, occupation, mental or physical activity and the normal weight in the adult.

There are bound to be differences in dietary practices in different parts of the world imposed by the various geographical, cultural and religious patterns. In this case it may be very difficult, inhumane and pure torture to restrict someone from eating his/her favourite dish, what he/she has been accustomed to from childhood or even from eating the only foodstuff that is available at any given moment. When and where necessary, restricted foods should be consumed in smaller quantities and at less regular intervals. What really matters is to complement the available restricted food with foodstuff that make up a balanced and healthy diet.

No matter one's status, creed, age, gender, culture or origin, one must never compromise vegetables, fruits, nuts and whole grains such as oats, cereals and brown rice. They have lots of fibre, vitamins and minerals and are known to have all the anti-oxidant and alkalinizing properties needed by the body.

A variety of spices such as ginger, turmeric, garlic cloves, cinnamon, etc. should be consumed also. They have potent anti-oxidant and anti-inflammatory effects on the body leading to various health benefits.

Probiotic foods such as yoghurt should be consumed often. They facilitate the activities of useful gut bacteria.

It is advisable to consume only natural and fresh fruit juice. Canned, packaged and ice-cold fruit juice with artificial preservatives should be shunned.

Minimal quantities of alcohol are needed by the body. Alcoholics are therefore cautioned to always drink with moderation.

Avoid doing drugs or indulging in smoking. They are addictive and can cause serious social and health hazards. Once addicted to them you cannot resist the urge to use them no matter the hazards they cause on your health. Drugs affect both the user and the people around him (family members, kids and even unborn babies). Same for smoking; it is bad for the smoker as well as those around him inhaling the smoke passively.

Commonly used drugs fall into the following main categories:

+Stimulants (eg cocaine).

+Depressants (eg alcohol).

+Narcotic analgesics or opioids (eg heroin).Tramadol falls under this category and it is a strong narcotic painkiller used to treat long-standing, excruciating pain where weaker painkillers have proved ineffective. It is supposed to be sold only on medical prescription but it is now known to be a major cause of destruction of our addicted youths due to illicit sales and purchases in our communities.

Smoking can cause respiratory tract diseases (especially lung cancer), premature aging, poor vision, stroke and coronary heart disease. During pregnancy, smoking increases the risk of preterm birth, low birth weight and some congenital anomalies of the mouth and lip. There is also an increased risk of Sudden Infant Death Syndrome (SIDS).

The best treatment for drug addiction is to prevent it. Our youths should be sensitized on the deleterious effects of drugs on their health and the health of those around them, especially their family members and loved ones. In the beginning the user wants to be bold and feel high. With time the functions of the brain begin to change and you may finally end up losing control, leading to damaging behaviour.

Children and young adults are advised to reduce the consumption of commercial sweets, as well as pastries and desserts rich in animal fats.

Eating cold foods should be avoided at all times and by all age groups. Vegetables should not be overwashed, overheated or overcooked.

Overfeeding should be discouraged; for it is not only unhealthy, but also sinful. It is gluttony! The Bible cautions that if you have a big appetite, restrain yourself (Prov. 23:2). Overeating causes a lot of havoc to your digestive system and this results in many health problems. The more food we eat, the more the energy needed for digestion. We then experience body weakness as a result.

'Grains (cereals), fruits, nuts and vegetables make up the food chosen for us by the creator'.

- Ellen G. White

2.2-1 HOW AND WHEN TO EAT

For better health benefits, it is very important to know when, how and what to eat.

<u>Breakfast</u>

Should be considered as the most important meal of the day and must never be compromised. It should be rich in foods that supply energy. In fact, the most appetising foods should be reserved for breakfast because it is the only time that heavy eating is justified. The time for breakfast should preferably be between 7:00am and 9:00am.

<u>Lunch</u>

Is a meal taken in the middle of the day (noon meal). It can be eaten in three courses: *a first course of energy foods, a second course of protein foods and a last course comprising a dessert.* Lunch should be eaten between 1:00pm and 3:00pm

Supper

Is the main evening meal. It should be taken between 5:00pm and 7:00pm. This supper time is very important because the human body is very inactive during sleep and the digestive system needs sufficient time to permit better assimilation of foods eaten during the day before one goes to bed at night. Supper is not always necessary for adults. It is good for children and those who perform intense physical activity. Not eating supper is indeed the best and surest way of losing weight. Abstaining from supper also improves on the quality of sleep. Where supper is needed, it should be light and should contain minimal fat. It can comprise of fresh fruits or fruit salad with crackers or whole wheat toast or with yoghurt, cottage cheese or vegetable dish.

A Snack is usually a small meal that is eaten between the main meals or a very small meal taken for lunch or supper.

The notion of having 'three square meals' a day is misguided, misconstrued, unhealthy and must be disregarded. I'm very much of the opinion that

A huge breakfast is laudable;

A huge lunch is pardonable;

But a huge supper is abominable.

This is consistent with the saying that; one should eat breakfast like a king, lunch like a prince and supper like a pauper.

Generally, it is unhealthy to eat between the main meals. Notwithstanding, if one must take something between meals, it is ideal to take fresh/dried fruits, nuts, fresh fruit juice or water. Always remember to take them fresh and not ice-cold. Also, the fruit juice or water should be taken on an empty stomach or at least 30 to 40 minutes before or after a main meal. It is worth noting that a snack is meant to be a very small meal and should not be taken in excess.

'Bad men live to eat and drink, whereas good men eat and drink in order to live'.

- Socrates

2.2-2 BABY NUTRITION

It would be incomplete and unfair to talk about healthy human feeding without discussing infant feeding. This forms the foundation of a healthy life in the life of a human being. From birth, babies should receive exclusive breast feeding. Exclusive breast feeding is when a baby receives only breast milk without any additional food or drink, not even water, until the age of about 06 months.

The baby can start receiving other foods at six months of age, such as vegetables, grains, fruits, proteins, etc. while continuing with breast milk until the age of one to two years, depending on the mother's decision. Exclusive breast feeding has the following health benefits:

☐ Breast milk is readily available and at the right composition and temperatures.

- It is very clean and has reduced risk of contamination.
- It lowers the baby's risk of having asthma or allergies.
- It increases resistance to infections, such as ear and respiratory tract infections and reduces bouts of diarrhoea in the baby.
- The baby ends up being relatively healthy and having fewer hospitalisations and trips to the doctor.
- It is financially advantageous as it is affordable to all mothers, irrespective of socio-economic standing.

Healthy feeding in humans therefore begins with

exclusive breast feeding in new born babies. However, it must be done under strict and proper hygienic conditions. The breast feeding mother must take good care of her breasts in general, and the nipples in particular, especially if some greedy husbands have to play with or even help the baby in sucking the breasts, notwithstanding the milk flow. The father's hands or mouth may leave some germs on the nipples in the process. This is even more imperative during this era of the Covid-19 pandemic, where preventive and other hygienic measures must be enforced at all levels.

2.2-3 PRAYING BEFORE AND AFTER MEALS

The spiritual aspect associated with eating and with good health is often overlooked or forgotten by so many people. We should always call on God, the provider, to bless each meal before eating, and also to thank him after eating for making it possible for us to be able to eat and enjoy the meal. We should be able to reap all the spiritual, healing and biological benefits from the food. There are many out there who have food but cannot eat, and many who can eat but have no food.

The opening prayer is widely known as '*Grace before meals*', and the closing prayer is referred to as '*Grace after meals*'. Although this happens to be a routine for most Christians, still many people either forget or are simply shy to say these prayers in gatherings or public places.

These prayers are also important in the sense that, they take care of any eventual evil or occultic manipulation on the food or drink we take into our bodies. Always remember that in all circumstances, we should give thanks to God. (1 Thess 5:18).

2.3 WATER INTAKE

We've already read the story of Daniel, how he and his three friends took water as the only complement to their vegetable diet. This confirms the vital role played by water in the human body. The popular slogan '*Water is life*', is supported by the fact that the human body is made up of about 70 per cent water (H_2O). Water is the most important nutrient for the human body. It plays a vital role in regulating body temperature, transporting nutrients and oxygen to cells, removing waste, cushioning joints and protecting organs and tissues.

The human body loses much water each day through perspiration, urination/stool and exhalation. The amount of drinking water varies. It depends on physical activity, age, health status and environmental conditions. People who live in a cool climate need less water intake than people who live in a warmer climate.

A normal adult needs to drink about 1.5 – 2 litres of water a day to prevent dehydration. Drinking fresh or warm water is healthy for the body, so we should avoid drinking cold or ice-cold water which is harmful to the organism.

The timing is also important. Drinking water at the right time maximises its effectiveness and health benefits. A glass of water should be taken first thing in the morning after waking up from sleep. Another glass of water should be taken about 30 minutes before having a bath. This is healthy for the cardio-vascular system and can lower one's blood pressure. Similar health benefits are obtained by taking a glass of water about 30 minutes before bed time.

It is also advisable to always keep drinking water close to your bed, so you can take a glass when you wake up at night and you feel thirsty. When you feel tired during the day, make sure you take at least a glass of water. Fatigue is one of the signs of dehydration. The same applies when one is ill; one should drink much water including other fluids like tea and fruit juice, in order to increase one's total intake.

Besides rehydrating the body, water helps to wash away germs and viruses. It also plays a vital role in dissolving calculi (gall bladder, kidney or bladder stones). Water should be taken between meals and not during meals; at least 30 to 40 minutes before or after meals. It prepares the stomach for food and cleans out any leftover tastes from earlier food, drinks or smoking, while waiting to have the next meal or snack.

Whenever one feels hungry and food is not ready or available, one should drink at least a glass of water. This is because water makes one feel full, thus sustaining one till food is readily available. You may even realise after taking the glass of water that you no longer need food, and this is because it was thirst, and not hunger, that was actually the problem.

Before and after a workout, it is advisable to drink water. This would protect against dehydration on the one hand, and replace fluids lost through perspiration and urination on the other hand. Hydration is also essential to guard against heatstroke in very hot places or frostbite caused by severe cold.

Avoid taking much water at once or in a haste because it may cause abdominal discomfort or cramps. As a general rule, much of the daily water intake should be during the day, and less at night. Water should not be taken only when one is thirsty, for it may not be sufficient to maintain proper or adequate hydration.

A dark-yellow urine is an indication that one hasn't taken enough water. On the other hand, a clear urine is an indication that one has taken enough water, for someone with normal kidney function and with no other related disease.

SOME TYPES OF WATER

Alkaline water is water with the pH above 7 and closer to 8.8. This makes it effective in neutralising excessive acids in the blood. It also gives the water an anti-oxidant and anti-aging effect.

Distilled water is pure and chemical free. It is the most pure toxin-free drink available and has no health risks associated. It contains no mineral salts such as calcium and potassium as in mineral water, and contains neither toxins nor germs. It is therefore perfectly suitable and recommended for human consumption.

Mineral water is water occurring in nature and derived mainly from springs. It contains some dissolved salts in it and is often bottled and sold as germ-free drinking water.

The choice, type and quantity of drinking water may depend on the climatic conditions, one's physical activity or occupation, the amount of oligo-elements in one's blood, the blood pH and one's socio-economic status. It is important to note that the best or recommended position for drinking water is the sitting or squatting position.

More health benefits can be derived from drinking warm or hot water. The Covid-19 pandemic has imposed this further. One can also derive more health benefits if squeezed fresh lemon juice is added to the warm or hot water, especially in the first glass of water taken in the morning after getting up from bed.

'Water is the only drink for a wise man'
                              - Henry David Thoreau

Like in eating, one should endeavour to pray always over the water before drinking, no matter the source. By praying to God in faith, one will be able to derive all the biological, healing and spiritual benefits from the water consumed.

We are reminded that, no matter what we're doing, even eating or drinking, we should do it all for the glory of God (1 Co 10:31). The same principle applies to urination and defecation, which are the end results of drinking and eating respectively. Many are those who are unable to urinate or defecate (urine or fecal retention) or who have no control over urination or defecation (urine or fecal incontinence). This is more than enough reason to pray and give thanks to God for those who, by His grace, can freely urinate or defecate without any inconveniences or difficulties. God is indeed worthy of our praises and we should give him thanks in everything.

2.4 EXERCISE AND PHYSICAL FITNESS

Aerobic and other fitness exercises should be done regularly. They make the heart, lung and muscles stronger and cause an increase in oxygen in the blood. This in turn keeps the body healthy and strong. It also improves on general fitness and reduces the risk of contracting many chronic diseases.

The frequency and type of exercise depends on the individual's age, gender, socio-economic status and state of health. Also, a combination of different types of exercises can provide more health benefits to an individual.

Endurance or aerobic activities increases one's breathing and heart rate. This helps to keep one's heart, lungs and circulatory system healthy, in addition to improving one's overall fitness. Examples of such exercises are ***brisk walking, jogging, swimming and biking.***

Energetic or resistance exercises make one's muscles stronger. Examples are weight lifting and stretching / pulling resistance bands or strings.

Balance exercises make it easy for one to walk on uneven surfaces without falling. An example of such exercises is practicing to stand on one leg or to stand on a pole.

Flexibility exercises help one to stretch one's muscles and assure easier and smoother movements of one's limbs. The practice of yoga, for example, makes one to be more flexible.

We should always try to select exercises that give us pleasure and a lot of fun doing them, so that things would be easier and better for us. Exercises should not be like a form of punishment or torture. We should also try to be safe, avoid injuries and avoid overdoing it.

A sedentary lifestyle should be vehemently

condemned because it involves little exercise or physical activity. People with a sedentary lifestyle are admonished to do more aerobic and other physical exercises at very regular intervals. To be strong and healthy, one must endeavour to walk more and drive less, and to stand more and sit less.

It is commonplace, nowadays, to find parents who are physically stronger and healthier than their children. This is because children of this generation are less involved in outdoor games, physical activities or long distance trekking, than their parents were in their youthful days. Children of today play more computer games, spend more time watching TV series or movies, and focus more on their laptops and android phones. They play less among themselves; they have no time to tell or narrate historic tales and other fascinating stories amongst themselves or within their families, and even avoid doing simple house chores.

This sedentary lifestyle and physical inactiveness makes them physically, mentally and emotionally unfit and less resistant to illness. It also makes them sluggish in their ways and decreases their general alertness and IQ (intelligence quotient). They should be made to understand that *all play and no work* makes one unhealthy and misfit in society.

Youths, as well as adults living such a sedentary lifestyle are exhorted to get out of slumber and engage in serious, frequent or regular aerobic and other physical exercises. This will greatly improve their overall health and fitness.

Couples who actively take part in regular, frequent and committed sexual intercourse make a physiologically, psychologically and emotionally stronger and healthier union. However, the duration, intensity and frequency of intercourse depend on the age and state of health of the spouses. At an advanced age, sexual intercourse should not be exaggerated or abusive, but must be done with moderation and care.

A pregnant woman with a normally evolving pregnancy must continue with her house chores and be involved in trekking and other physical activities, even during the last 3 months of gestation.

Throughout pregnancy, aerobic exercises and other physical activities make both mother and foetus healthy, facilitate the progression of labour and eases delivery. Our mothers and grandmothers used to do the chores, do farm work and even split wood right up to the days preceding delivery; an example worth emulating by our wives, sisters and daughters of this generation.

The so-called emancipated or wealthy women of today, who love to be pampered, petted or carried all over the house during pregnancy by their darling husbands, should desist from inertness and physical inactivity during the gestational period. It may account for some cases of difficult deliveries or stillbirths. However, when there are threats of an abortion, miscarriage or preterm delivery, rest is indicated and sexual intercourse proscribed.

2.4 - 1   DIET AND PHYSICAL EXERCISE

Eating and exercise go hand in hand and it is good to control how, when and what to eat when exercising.

Carbohydrates are necessary for maximum energy. Large meals should be eaten at least 3 to 4 hours before exercising. Small meals or snacks should be taken 1 to 3 hours before exercising.

The tendency is for one to feel sluggish if one eats too much before an exercise. Eating too little before a workout would not give one enough energy to carry on.

Water intake is very important because the body needs to be well-hydrated when exercising; and water is the best way to replace lost fluids through perspiration and sweating. However, those involved in competitive sports or games may need a sports drink that would help maintain their body's electrolyte balance and give them a bit more energy, because of the carbohydrate contained in the sports drink.

Eating or drinking, as mentioned above, before exercising, can improve work out performance and may enable one to workout for a longer duration or intensity. Not eating or drinking may make one feel sluggish or light-headed. The athlete doing marathon needs more energy than the person engaged in a short distance walk or jogging.

2.4 - 2   SPIRITUALITY AND PHYSICAL FITNESS

There exists a healthy and worthy relationship between spirituality and physical fitness. Physical exercises or activities keep the body lean, fit and strong to do one's everyday spiritual practices. A healthy body will prompt or enable one to live out a spiritual life filled with action, integrity, faith and hope.

The practice of Yoga is one of the most popular spiritual exercises as evidenced by the Hindu religion. It connects the mind, body and soul, and can improve on one's flexibility, strength, cardio-pulmonary fitness, alertness of the mind, mood and overall life. It enhances and improves on one's spiritual health as well.

Exercises also boost the brain's mental energy, thus enhances meditation, gratitude, appreciation, connection with nature and love of neighbour. This gets us connected to God our creator as a result.

Hinduism and other Asian religions are known and acknowledged for their physical exercises and activities that are related to their beliefs and spirituality.

Christians, either consciously or unconsciously, also practice certain physical exercises that boost their spirituality; such as standing, sitting, kneeling, genuflecting, raising of hands, closing of eyes, bowing, prostrating, clapping of hands, singing and dancing. These practices, if observed strictly and reverently as prescribed by the Church, would cause an improvement in our mental, physical and spiritual health, as well as our connectivity to God. These exercises or activities also play a non-negligible role in keeping those who happen to dose off during worship awake and focused. Those who may have restrictions or exemptions from these practices during worship are the sick and elderly.

Fasting, besides nourishing one's spirituality, can enable one lose weight, improve on one's insulin sensitivity and reduce oxidative stress in the body. It can also help in regulating one's hormone levels, thus reducing one's appetite and causing one to eat only when hungry. Fasting enables the body to heal itself and also gives the gut time to relax. Fasting for about 3-6 days is beneficial to our health, and can cause a reduction or disappearance of flatulence, indigestion, constipation and headaches. It is ironical to break your fast by overfeeding. On the contrary, small portions of food should be taken in 3-4 hourly intervals after breaking your fast, in order to regulate the functioning of the digestive system to its original state.

2.5 ENOUGH REST AND SLEEP.

2.5-1 SLEEP

Sleep is a naturally recurring state of mind and body, characterised by altered consciousness, relatively inhibited sensory activity, inhibition of nearly all voluntary muscles and reduced interactions with surroundings (Wikipedia).

Sleep happens to be a vital indicator of overall health and wellbeing. Our age and lifestyle affect the quality and quantity of sleep. To obtain optimum health, a good sleep is necessary and this can affect hormone levels, mood and weight of an individual.

Sleep and death have a very close relationship but for the fact that during sleep one's heart continues to function and the pulse is palpable. A great literary icon pondered this relationship and wrote:

'Sleep may be the image or brother of death, for in sleep the body rests while the soul remains awake, so in death the body rests while the soul and the spirit live.'

- William Shakespeare

We spend about one third of our lives sleeping. The natural sleep/wake cycle (circadian rhythm) can be interrupted by certain stimulants, such as energy drinks, coffee and various forms of light and sounds. Common sleep problems include snoring, sleep apnoea, insomnia, sleep deprivation and restless leg syndrome.

Healthy sleep habits can significantly improve on one's quality of life. And it is advisable to stick to a sleep schedule of the same bedtime and the same wake up time. This helps to regulate the body's clock.

'Early to bed and early to rise makes a man healthy, wealthy and wise.'

- Benjamin Franklin

The health benefits derived from sleep depends on the number of hours invested in sleep per night. Healing, recovery and rebuilding take place during a good quality sleep. Those who have difficulties sleeping at night should avoid having a nap during the day.

A good night's sleep of eight (08) full hours would keep an adult healthy, fresh and strong enough to face a new day. A normal adult should go to bed by 9 to 10pm and wake up by 5 to 6am.

The requisite numbers of hours of sleep increases with decreasing age; babies need more hours of sleep than adults, ranging from 14 to 17 hours (newborn) to 7 to 9 hours (adults).

To enable quality sleep, one needs to sleep on a comfortable mattress and pillows, on clean bed clothes and in a cool bedroom that is free from noise and light. One can use certain devices such as ear plugs, curtains and eye shades to prevent noise and light accordingly.

Sleep positions may vary according to one's

predilection, age or health condition. It is safer to sleep on your back than on your belly, and better to sleep on your left side of the body than on your right side. When lying on your left side, there is better blood flow and lymphatic drainage. Mothers are advised to desist from putting their babies to sleep lying on their bellies; it may result in sudden death, referred to as crib death or cot death.

It is unhealthy to get up from bed abruptly or in a hurry after waking up from sleep. It should be a gradual and well-coordinated process in order to avoid or reduce sudden death.

A three times half minute (one and a half minutes) wake-up procedure can reduce or avoid sudden death in those who get up, especially at night, to urinate, answer a phone call, or in reaction to a sudden sound or imminent danger. The procedure is as follows:

☐ *When you wake up, stay lying in bed for the first half minute (30 seconds)*

☐ *Then, sit up in bed for the next half minute (30 seconds)*

☐ *Lastly, turn sideways and sit on the edge of the bed with your legs lowered, for the last half minute (30 seconds), after which you can now stand up and move.*

This simple but life-saving '***one and a half minute (90 seconds)***' exercise will help avoid or reduce the risk of having a stroke or cardiac arrest, thus minimising the possibility of one falling or of sudden death. And this may happen to anybody, irrespective of age, gender, creed or socio-economic status. Therefore, no matter the urgency or impending danger that may cause you to wake up from your sleep, always remember to be calm and follow the above 'one and a half minute' prescription. The rest should be put under God's care; 'For He is our shelter and our strength, always ready to help in times of trouble (Ps 43:1).'

He also exhorts us to be still and know that He is God (Ps 46:10). Again, science and religion are in perfect harmony here, without any contradiction or rivalry.

2.5-2 ENOUGH REST

Regardless of one's career or preoccupation, it is imperative for one to take some time off and rest. This can be done daily, weekly, monthly or yearly depending on one's activity, job description, age or health status.

Even God the Father rested after creating the world. It is written that by the seventh day God had finished what he had been doing and stopped working (Gen 2:2). In this case he rested after one full week of divine work.

We know of workaholics who spend all their time working without any rest, break or holiday. They fail to realise that if they happen to crack up, collapse, have a stroke or die because of unending work demands, they would sooner or later be replaced by others. Work must continue and life must go on, regardless of the regrettable demise or incapacity of a hardworking and lovable colleague or employee.

Taking a break or having some rest refreshes one's memory (improves alertness) and makes one stronger and more productive in the execution of one's duties or assignments. Also, retreating from bustle and hustle of worldly activities and moving to a quiet environment to rest, or meditating on God's word and communicating one-on-one with Him in prayer, will nourish and prepare one spiritually to face the world with all its trials and tribulations, as well as one's work demands or exigencies. It is documented that our Lord Jesus himself withdrew to a lonely place to pray to God the Almighty Father (Lk 5:16).

It is worth mentioning that it is very unhealthy and unproductive to spend more time resting or sleeping and less or no time working. Rest should be well deserved.

'The sleep of a labouring man is sweet'.   - **Ecclesiastes.**

2.6 HAPPINESS, LAUGHTER, ANGER AND FORGIVENESS.

2.6-1 HAPPINESS/LAUGHTER
' When things are going well for you, be glad and

when trouble comes, just remember: God sends both happiness and trouble; you never know what is going to happen next'. **(Ecc 7:14)**

We should endeavour to be happy at all times because both good and bad times come from God. Whatever happens to us happens according to His will and no mortal being can be certain about what the future may bring. We are expected to be joyful always, pray at all times and be thankful in all circumstances (1 Thess 5:16-18).

There is the popular saying that, *'laughter is the best medicine'*. It produces a lot of health benefits such as pain relief (analgesic effect), good quality sleep, improved digestion, enhancing happiness, easing tension, invigorating the body, combating stress, reducing blood pressure, boosting the immune system and increasing one's self confidence.

'Laughter is a tranquiliser with no side effects'.
- Arnold Glasgow

2.6-2 ANGER / FORGIVENESS

*'Holding on to anger is like drinking poison
and expecting the other person to die.'*
- **Buddha**

Contrary to laughter, anger is known to be a great killer. It causes inner pressure, inner heat, inner pain, evil thoughts, grudges and thoughts of vengeance. A violent outburst of anger may cause cerebral-vascular accidents leading to stroke and death.

Anger is not only unhealthy and harmful to the individual, but also to persons around him/her. The Scripture cautions us not to make friends with people who have hot, violent tempers (Prov 22: 24). It also reminds us to be quick to listen, but slow to become angry and that man's anger does not achieve God's righteous purpose (Jas 1:19-20).

One of the best and practical ways to vent out anger or hurt is to cry and shed tears. Do not hold back tears when the occasion arises. Let them flow down your cheeks till you're able to calm down and dry them off. The slang 'crocodile tears' is used when someone is faking to be hurt or in pain, and is shedding tears, when actually he/she is not in pain or in distress. In reality, the crocodile doesn't shed tears as a result of pain, but in order to maintain a physiological balance.

After the death of his friend Lazarus, Jesus shed tears. This happens to be the shortest verse in the bible; *'And Jesus wept'* (Jn 11:35). It was true that Jesus was touched by the death of his friend Lazarus, but the main reason for his weeping was to ease an inner pain and disappointment that emanated from the fact that he was disgusted by so much blindness and lack of faith by those who were around.

Shedding of tears or weeping should therefore not

always be considered as a sign of weakness or desperation. It is also necessary for emotional balance and wellbeing.

We are admonished to get rid of all bitterness, passion and anger. That, there should be no more shouting or insults and no more hateful feelings of any sort. And instead, we should be kind and tender-hearted to one another as God has forgiven us through Christ (Eph 4:31-32). Forgiveness has great healing properties. It is of utmost importance to always free yourself from self-imprisonment by forgiving all those who wrong or hurt you. This will make you feel happier, freer, better and healthier.

'To forgive is to gain victory over the enemy'

- Hazrat Ali

The spiritual importance of forgiveness is stated in the 'Lord's prayer' thus: 'if you forgive others the wrongs they have done to you, your Father in heaven will also forgive you. But if you do not forgive others, then your father will not forgive the wrongs you have done'. (Mtt 6:14-15)

'To err is human, to forgive divine'

- Alexander Pope

We should try, no matter the hurt or pain, to forgive one another for as many times as we hurt or inflict pain on one another. And this forgiveness should be elastic, having no limits as to the number of times one forgives. This point was made crystal clear by Jesus Christ when he exhorted Peter and his disciples to forgive, not seven times, but seventy times seven (Mtt 18:21-22). As we continue to do this, we continue to release, neutralise or completely efface the pressure, tension and suffocation inside us, as a result of bearing grudges.

Forgiveness is the surest way to disarm someone who wrongs you and it paves the way for love to prevail and, eventually, for peace to reign.

Also, the craving for vengeance is suppressed if we forgive. Our Lord Jesus warns us not to take revenge on someone who wrongs us; that if anyone slaps you on the right cheek, let him slap your left cheek too (Mtt 5:39). *'Do not take revenge on anyone or continue to hate him/her, but love your neighbour as you love yourself. I am the Lord.'*

- (Lev 19:18)

2.7   IMPROVE ON HUMAN RELATIONS

Improving on one's relations with other people,

especially family members, friends, colleagues, neighbours and the community, is based on love. He who gives love will receive love in return and consequently will be free, healthy and live happily ever after.

> *'All human relations untouched by love take place in the dark'.*

> **- Richard Rorty**

Our Lord Jesus summarised the greatest of all commandments as follows:

"'Love **the Lord your God with all your heart, with all your soul and with all your mind**!' This is the greatest and most important commandment. The second most important commandment is like it: '**Love your neighbour as you love yourself**.' The whole Law of Moses and the teachings of the prophets depend on these two commandments (Mtt 22:37-39)."

Of the three most important virtues; faith, hope and love, the greatest of them is said to be love (1 Co 13:13).

It is also said that, love is patient and kind; it is not jealous or conceited or proud (1 Co 13:14). We are therefore admonished to live and show love in both the vertical (to God) and horizontal (to fellow humans) components of our lives. This would ensure perfect health in mind, body and soul.

Love is the first step towards forgiveness and reconciliation in the sense that, if you must forgive anyone who wrongs you, then you must start by loving that person.

'Hate stirs up trouble, but love overlooks all offences'

- Prov 10:12

We can always show kindness by being charitable and good to others in our everyday interactions with one another. In a bid to socialize, we try to spend valuable time out of our busy schedule with friends, family members or neighbours, in order to have mutual enjoyment. This may be in the form of sporting activities, cultural activities, having a common meal or participating in other forms of entertainment in the community. It could be very refreshing and invigorating, and it could help reduce or prevent certain stress-related ailments and other psychosomatic illnesses. It makes one to know, accept and understand other people better and to develop trust and self-confidence.

The Covid-19 pandemic has re-awakened the undisputed need for mankind to love and care for one another. Wherever we find ourselves, we should endeavour to be an advocate of peace and promoter of justice and, without fear or favour, endeavour to be the voice of the voiceless. Being at peace with oneself and with one another would go a long way in enhancing our individual and collective health.

2.8   HAVE JOB SATISFACTION AND SECURITY

'Work because you want to, not because you have to'

- Mike Mc, Clary

For longevity and wellness to be achieved, one must avoid stressful jobs that have no job security. This is because one's income may change negatively or one may be laid off at any time, with or without notice. Your job doesn't guarantee financial security and freedom. These can only be guaranteed if one discovers and exploits his/her individual talents and passions positively, for a better livelihood.

'We can create the ultimate job security by becoming less dependent on the organization for which we work and more dependent on our own resources.'

- Bo Bennett

To be successful and financially secure, one should strive to be an entrepreneur instead of an employee, or an employee engaged in some entrepreneurial activities that would fetch extra income. According to the Psalmist, 'your work will provide for your needs, and you will be happy and prosperous (Ps 128:2).'

As a youth, I was cautioned by my elder brother, a priest, that if I choose to do anything for a living, I should make sure it comes from my heart, and that whatever I do in life, I should endeavour to do it well and with love. Thanks to him, I live and work based on those principles he inculcated in me. To God be the glory!

In order to be happy and in good health, one should love one's job or preoccupation, and especially enjoy the fruits of one's labour.

'All of us should eat and drink, and enjoy what we have worked for. It is God's gift. **(Eccl 3:13)**

2.9 TIMELY RESPONSE TO NATURE'S CALL

Substances no longer useful to the human body have to be disposed of by way of nature's call. The most common ways are by urination, defecation and farting, with the release of urine, faeces and gas, respectively.

Once these substances are ready to be disposed of by the human body, certain warning signals are received by the body according to the type of substance or organ involved. Once this happens, one should not resist the urge to urinate, defecate or fart at the appropriate moment.

Same principle applies to coughing out sputum or clearing of catarrh from one's throat or nose, respectively. One must not try to hold them back or swallow them. If one tries to swallow them, germs that are otherwise normal in the respiratory tract may find themselves in the gastro-intestinal tract where they may become harmful or pathogenic.

An overactive bladder causes frequent urination and it is very frustrating to wake up constantly late at night to go to the bathroom. Alcohol, caffeine, and some fruits such as water melon, pineapple and asparagus are natural diuretics that cause frequent urination. The consumption of these natural diuretics should be avoided or reduced after 5-7pm, in order to avoid getting up from bed at night constantly to answer nature's call.

Keeping urine in a full bladder for too long may facilitate the progression of urinary tract infections (UTI). It may also cause rupture of the bladder in the unfortunate occurrence of a road traffic accident, or any other traumatic incident like fighting, assault or contact sporting activities. Also, resisting the urge to defecate or fart may cause serious abdominal discomfort.

Patients with pelvic masses or other pathological conditions that cause faecal/urinary retention or faecal/urinary incontinence are advised to seek immediate medical attention.

When it comes to farting, we should endeavour to tolerate and bear with one another, no matter how smelly, messy or explosive it may be.

2.10 SAVOUR NATURE

Spending time savouring nature can be a powerful tool for self-reflection and personal health.

Walking among trees, walking on a sandy beach, hearing the sounds of birds, feeling the wind blowing on your face and body, climbing on hilltops and observing exotic vegetation and spectacular scenery etc. are some of the ways by which we can enjoy nature positively.

Spending some quiet moment in nature improves one's self-discipline, refreshes one's memory and activates all the sensory organs. It improves on the overall physical health and it also uplifts one's spirituality.

2:11 HYGIENE AND SANITATION.

PREVENTION IS BETTER THAN CURE!!

Generally, hygiene and sanitation is the practice of keeping oneself and one's surroundings clean in a bid to prevent infection and disease, in order to remain healthy and fit. Its ultimate goal is to maintain good health and increase our lifespans.

Besides its importance in assuring physical, psychological, social and spiritual health, personal hygiene also contributes to the socio-economic development of the society.

Sanitation deals with latrines and proper waste disposal, amongst others.

The most important personal hygiene practice is washing of hands. It helps prevent illness and infection from bacteria or viruses and is an effective way to harness the spread of germs. This explains its pivotal role in the prevention of COVID-19.

Proper washing of hands is done as follows:
- wet hands with clean water and apply soap
- lather hands by rubbing thoroughly with soap
- scrub hands for at least 20seconds
- rinse hands well with running water
- dry hands with clean towel or air-dry.

Other personal hygienic measures involve: caring for your nails; cleaning your teeth ; clearing ear wax; showering every day; washing of hair about three times a week; getting rid of bad breath; using natural deodorants; cleaning the feet and protecting the skin from excessive sun. We should also endeavour to use clean towels, clean underpants, clean dresses and sleep on clean bed clothes.

Overall, good personal hygiene not only benefits your own health but directly Impacts the lives of those around you .It is also spiritually beneficial, for "cleanliness is next to godliness."

2.12 LIVE ONE DAY AT A TIME

'So, do not worry about tomorrow; it will have enough worries of its own. There is no need to add to the troubles each day brings...'   **(Mtt 6:34)**

To worry makes one unhappy and frightened. It makes one uncertain about future happenings and creates a lot of anxiety or sleeplessness. This may lead to psychosomatic disorders or other unpleasant health conditions.

Fretting unnecessarily about the future pushes some of us into criminal activities such as stealing, corruption, extortion, scamming, embezzlement, prostitution, falsehood and lies telling. Some people live above their means and others amass much wealth in a bid to procuring enough provisions and property for future generations. Only God sees into and knows the future, so it would be absurd and foolhardy for people to spend their time trying to procure property or money for future generations.

Jesus said to a crowd he was teaching; 'Watch out and guard yourselves from every kind of greed; because a person's true life is not made up of the things he owns, no matter how rich he may be (Lk 12:15).' Also, God said to a rich man who had stored enough crops and goods that would last him so many years; 'You fool! This very night you will have to give up your life; then who will get all these things you have kept for yourself?' (Lk 12:20).

The best investment in this world to cater for future generations is to invest in your children by educating them or teaching them a trade; not necessarily to leave them much property. They too will invest in their own children, who will in turn invest in their own children and the chain would continue for generations upon generations to come. That would go a long way in reducing unnecessary stress as experienced by many parents today, and consequently would improve on their health, integrity and longevity. We are admonished to be wise enough not to wear ourselves out trying to get rich (Prov 23:4), for it will obviously take a toll on our health.

All we need as we journey through this earth is our daily bread, just enough for us and our basic needs. Our Lord highlighted this point when he taught his disciples how to pray, saying: 'Give us today the food we need (Mtt

6:11).' He did not teach us to ask God to give us tomorrow or in the future, the food we need. Tomorrow or the future will surely take care of itself, if only we believe and have faith in Him. Food here may mean money, property, etc.

2.13 PREPARE ADEQUATELY FOR RETIREMENT

Mankind must work hard in order to have food, shelter, clothing and other basic requirements for survival.

At the beginning of creation, after the disobedience of man, God said; 'You will have to work hard all your life to make it (the soil) produce enough food for you (Gen 3:17b).' Today, besides farming, work comprises various professions, careers or vocations. By working, we can plan or provide for our families and effectively earn a comfortable living. If we live within our means and manage our hard-earned income properly and responsibly, we don't need to steal, extort, embezzle or misappropriate funds in order to procure wealth and property for future generations.

Due to advanced age or incapacity, one is bound to retire from work by giving up one's regular work, profession, career or vocation. The age of retirement varies according to the type of assignment, duty or profession and according to the country in which one retires. It said that age is just a number, but retirement is one of the greatest gifts to mankind. It is a time to enjoy the things you never could enjoy before.

Due to ill-health, incapacity or for other reasons which may be purely personal, one may also leave work on voluntary retirement, even before the official retirement age.

Generally, retirement should not be seen as a punitive measure or as an end to one's active or productive life. It isn't the end of the road, but just a turn in the road. It enables one to rest after a befitting career, or to enable one engage in a less demanding or less stressful job. In some cases, depending on one's activity or strategic planning, one can even make more money in the retirement period. Never say never! It is a period when you have to enjoy a new chapter in your life, especially enjoying being your own boss.

If one decides to go on voluntary retirement due to job dissatisfaction, it will open up opportunities for one to have a job with better conditions in terms of job satisfaction or better wages.

The time to start preparing for retirement is from when one starts working. Instead of being carried away by youthful exuberance and bad peer pressure, one should start planning for one's family and for a home from the early stages of one's productive life. One should never think of waiting for retirement before building a house or making a family. Some parents put all their hopes on their children to provide all their basic needs, provisions, including building them a house, when they retire. It may be suicidal for such parents if the children end up disappointing them. It would be a plus and a blessing to have children who would be willing to help you alleviate your problems, both financially and materially, at this stage in your life. Such children too would, in turn, be rewarded abundantly by God Almighty.

It is advisable to trim your family size according to your capacities and means. Do not give birth to children you'd not be able to take care of. Always have it in mind that children are a gift from God and parents are mere caretakers here on earth. It is the parents' primary responsibility to take good care of them and guide them on the right path till they become independent.

In Western countries, there are old peoples' homes to take care of people who are too old, weak or ill to be able to cater for themselves. In countries where these facilities don't exist, people must prepare adequately for retirement and old age. It is also advisable, where possible, to have some side assets, besides one's pension, that would help in sustaining one throughout retirement up until death. No matter how old one is, provided one is still alive, he or she would need food, drinks, medications and some money to pay bills and partake in some social, family and church contributions.

Adequate planning in anticipation for retirement would enable one experience a safe, secure and fun-filled retirement. In some developed countries, the citizens have social security as part of their retirement plan. Not preparing adequately for retirement may lead to misery, poverty, disappointment, abandonment or premature death. One can prepare for retirement emotionally or mentally by preparing about 1-5years in advance, thinking about what to do in retirement (a hobby or other interests), having it in mind that it is a process, discovering your new identity and purpose in life, certain goals to attain and by replacing work routine with new routines. Under normal circumstances, one should be able to enjoy an honest, happy, healthy and fulfilled life as one prepares for the last days. Every retiree's dream should be to have a well-deserved and happy retirement. After a long and successful career, one should be able to enjoy recreational activities that do not require much physical exertion or cause unhealthy exhaustion, but rather beneficial to the retiree's health. Examples of such activities are walking on a beach, travelling in a cruise ship, visiting various touristic attractions, etc. Some retirees spend valuable time being anxious about death, instead of focusing their gaze, thoughts and activities on living joyfully and healthily. At this stage in life, one should be reconciled with God and contemplate on life after death; for death is the inevitable end of all mankind. The choice of where and how to spend eternity depends on the individual; for salvation is said to be personal.

'There is no cure for birth and death, save to enjoy the interval.'

- George Santayana

PART THREE

DIE HAPPY

How you die is
quite important
but, by far more
important is, how
you live

- J.P, Vaswani

3:1   DEATH

'The goal of all life is death.'

- Sigmund Frend

Death is defined simply as the end of life; the total and permanent cessation of all the vital functions of an organism. (**Merriam Webster**)

According to plato, it is the end of terrestrial life and access to an ideal world. The Scriptures tell us that, when we die, our bodies will return to the dust of the earth, and the breath of life will go back to God, who gave it to us. (Eccl 12:7).

Every human being unconsciously practises how to die during sleep, like an athlete warming up for an Olympic race. In fact, the inactiveness or unconsciousness during sleep is a foretaste of death. The main difference is that sleep lasts only for a moment, with our pulses and breath intact. The reverse is true for death, which is a journey of no return, with an irreversible cessation of circulatory and respiratory functions.

We get up from sleep each day, mentally refreshed and physically invigorated, ready to go about our daily activities without knowing when, how and where we shall die. However, we should be aware that, the day of the

Lord will come as a thief comes at night (1 Thess 5:2). Many of us do not even contemplate on God's purpose for creating us. We just go on living each new day taking many things for granted, going about our daily preoccupations, chasing after things of the flesh and seeking power, fame and wealth. We forget that our main focus should be heaven-bound, not earth-bound.

Our basic Christian doctrine teaches us that, the reason why God made us is to KNOW him, LOVE him and SERVE him in this world, and be HAPPY with him forever in the next. Whatever we say or do in our lives, should be to His glory.

To live a purposeful life on earth, according to God's plan, we must anticipate death and ponder about how and where we would like to spend eternity. We are all destined to die.

'Seventy is the sum of our years, or eighty if we are strong, and most of them are fruitless toil, for they pass quickly and we drift away!' (Ps 90:10)

Death is part of life and should not be regarded as a separate entity or diametrically opposed to life. If we consider life to be an imaginary line, birth is at one extreme (1st part of that line) and death at the other extreme (last point). If the 1st part of this line (birth) is normal, the last point (death) cannot and should not be considered abnormal.

Death is therefore non-negotiable and nobody born of a woman is spared. Even Jesus Christ, who was both God and man was born of a woman, died as man and resurrected and ascended into heaven as the Son of man (God).

'Not only is death inevitable, death is necessary for us to inherit the new life we are to enjoy in Christ.'

- Max Lucado

Even on our dying beds, our faith should always be profound and unshakable. The Lord says; *'Be faithful to me, even if it means death, and I will give you life as your prize of victory'*. **(Rev. 2:10[b])**

3.2 DYING HAPPY IN FAITH

To die happy means being happy at the point of death. (This should not be mistaken for "to die happily", meaning being happy to die. A normal human being cannot be happy to die.) Faith makes death peaceful, acceptable and bearable.

When a person is terminally ill, or has attained a ripe old age, faith makes him/her more courageous and better prepared to welcome or accept death. When our time comes, let us be able to say like St Paul; *'As for me, the hour has come for me to be sacrificed; the time is here for me to leave this life. I have done my best in the race; I have run the full distance, and I have kept the faith'.* (2 Tim 4:6-7). We must prepare for the end and the only way to secure a place in God's kingdom is to persevere in faith and obey his laws and ordinances.

Faith also encourages, consoles, strengthens and prepares the minds of the family members and loved ones of the deceased. It is consoling to know that, although we may experience suffering and pain, this temporary trouble will only bring us tremendous and eternal glory, much greater than the trouble itself (2 Co 4:17).

Like the aged Simeon in the Bible, if we live on earth fully, faithfully and purposefully, according to God's plan, we should be able to embrace death in peace and say to the Lord; 'Now master, you are letting your servant go in peace as you promised' (Lk 2:29).

To die happy, we must learn to surrender all our pains, sufferings and afflictions to our Lord who said; *'Come to me all you who labour and are overburdened, and I will give you rest' Shoulder my yoke and learn from me for I am gentle and humble in heart and you will find rest for your souls'* (Mtt 11:19)

This applies to both the dying person (deceased) and members of his/her family, or loved ones (bereaved). Although it is normal and natural for them to be saddened and weep for the dying person or the deceased, they should accept the will of God and have hope that he/she will attain eternal life and be in perfect peace in the Lord's bosom. The scripture tells us that it is a foolish mistake to think that righteous people die and that their death is a terrible evil. That they leave us is not a disaster; in fact, the righteous are at peace. (Wis 3:2-3)

Those who live by faith with the hope of gaining eternal life will die happy.

3.3 ETERNITY

'There is no death, only a change of worlds.'

- Seattle

We are all pilgrims here on earth, passing from one life to another, and it is only through death that this obligatory and unavoidable transition is made possible. While life on earth is short-lived, life after death is believed to be eternal or everlasting.

In reality, it was not God's original plan for humans to die when He created the world. It was the Devil's jealousy that brought death into the world and those who belong to the devil are the ones who will die (Wis 2:23-24). It is therefore a matter of choice or free will; we are either in God's camp and thereafter enjoy eternal life, or choose to dine with the devil all our lives and thereafter suffer eternal damnation.

Living by faith makes a more profound meaning when we put it in the context of eternity.

Those who believed, trusted, hoped and who persevered in their faith, through thick and thin, during their lifetime on earth, are the ones to whom the Lord would say on judgement day; *'Come you that are blessed by my Father! Come and possess the kingdom which has been prepared for you ever since the creation of the world'.* (Mtt 25:34).

To those who had no faith, who lived contrary to the teachings of Christ, and who dined with the devil all their lives, the Lord would say; *'Away from me, you that are under God's curse! Away, to the eternal fire that has been prepared for the devil and his angels!'* (Mtt 25:41)

We are exhorted not to love the world or anything that belongs to the world. The world and everything in it that people desire is passing away, but those who do the will of God live forever (1Jn 2:15-17).

The ultimate goal of all humans is to gain eternal life. It is written; 'Will people gain anything if they win the whole world but lose their life? Of course not! There is nothing they can give to regain their life.' (Mtt 16:26)

'The Father loves His Son and has put everything in his power. Whoever believes in the Son has eternal life; whoever disobeys the Son will not have life, but will remain under God's punishment.'

- Jn 3:35-36

CONCLUSION

"What matters is not to add years to your

life but to add life to your years."

-Alexis.

The Medico-Scriptural Basis of Healing, Good Health and Dying Happy, as presented in this book ,can be summarized as follows:

+Live a life of UNWAVERING FAITH and have childlike trust and hope in God, your creator.

+Eat the RIGHT FOODS in the RIGHT PROPORTIONS and at the RIGHT TIME.

+Drink MUCH WATER during the day and AWAY FROM MEALS.

+Engage in frequent and regular AEROBIC and PHYSICAL/ENERGY EXERCISES.

+Do REGULAR MEDICAL CHECKUP and strive as much as possible to undergo HOLISTIC HEALING when sick or afflicted.

+Avoid STRESS and ANGER; LAUGH, LOVE and FORGIVE always.

+Have QUALITY SLEEP and ENOUGH REST.

+Make time to SAVOUR NATURE, to engage in SOCIAL ACTIVITIES and improve on HUMAN RELATIONS.

+Love whatever you do for a living, have JOB SATISFACTION and PREPARE ADEQUATELY for RETIREMENT.

+Live according to GOD'S PURPOSE and WILL for your life; keep His LAWS and ORDINANCES.

Observe these divinely inspired principles and enjoy a Healthy, Happy, Purposeful, Productive and Fulfilled Life, here on Earth and for Eternity. This is one area where RELIGION and SCIENCE are in Perfect HARMONY and doesn't in any way contradict one another.

The way to go about all these is by being Heavenly-bound, being focused on the set goals, having a positive mindset and to apply a lot of CONSISTENCY and SELF-DISCIPLINE.

At the end of it all, however hard we try, it is by the GRACE OF GOD that we can effectively achieve our objectives, for Life and Death are all in God's Hands.

To God be the GLORY.

REFERENCES

- http:// jean hails.org.au>health-a-z>nat.
- http:// medium.com>how-to-us.
- http:// www.breastfeeding-problems.com
- http:// www.care 2.com>greenliving>1.....
- http:// www.health fitness revolution.com
- http://www.healthline.com/nutrition/27-health-and nutrition-tips #section 7
- http:// www.sleepfoundation.org>health
- http:// www.what christians want to know.com
- http:// www.webmd.com>balance>guide
- http:// www.sleepfoundation.org>health ......
- Jabel D'cruz(2008). The best proverbs and Quotes.
- The Catholic Catechism (2008). For the Bamenda Ecclesiastical Province. (Based on the Catechism of the Catholic Church).
- The Good News Bible (1994). 2nd Edition.
- Picture quotes.com
- QuotesHD.com
- Retirementtipsandtricks.com>how_t.
- www.naturesleep.com>blog>thre..